José Roberto Cunha Lima
Maria Janete Gomes Ribeiro

Green Banana Flour Cookie

José Roberto Cunha Lima
Maria Janete Gomes Ribeiro

Green Banana Flour Cookie

Green banana flour cookie: An alternative for people with celiac disease

Imprint
Any brand names and product names mentioned in this book are subject to trademark, brand or patent protection and are trademarks or registered trademarks of their respective holders. The use of brand names, product names, common names, trade names, product descriptions etc. even without a particular marking in this work is in no way to be construed to mean that such names may be regarded as unrestricted in respect of trademark and brand protection legislation and could thus be used by anyone.

Cover image: www.ingimage.com

This book is a translation from the original published under ISBN 978-620-2-19533-1.

Publisher:
Sciencia Scripts
is a trademark of
Dodo Books Indian Ocean Ltd. and OmniScriptum S.R.L publishing group

120 High Road, East Finchley, London, N2 9ED, United Kingdom
Str. Armeneasca 28/1, office 1, Chisinau MD-2012, Republic of Moldova, Europe
Printed at: see last page
ISBN: 978-620-7-30555-1

SUMMARY

I would like to dedicate this to my dear family, made up of Maria Geonilde Gomes de Oliveira Amaro (mother), Gilson Ribeiro Amaro (father), Miria Gomes Ribeiro (sister) and Mateus Gomes Ribeiro (brother), for always believing and trusting in me, and who, regardless of any problem or difficulty, have been by my side, supporting me and believing that I am capable.

To my advisor José Roberto da Cunha Lima, for all the encouragement he has given me and for awakening in me an interest in research and not stopping here.

ACKNOWLEDGMENTS

First of all to God, who was my greatest safe haven, my everything, who gave me all the courage I needed to go beyond my limits during these four years dedicated to Nutrition and didn't let me lack the strength to achieve my goals. Thank you Lord for your immense grace!

To my parents Maria Geonilde and Gilson, who are responsible for every step forward in my life. Throughout all these years, you have been my greatest example of strength, courage and perseverance, so that I will never give up in the face of the first obstacle. You will always be my great example of victory. Thank you for everything, I love you very much.

To my siblings Miria and Mateus, for all their support and patience and for always supporting me in all my choices, and that I know I can always count on. I love you all.

Many thanks to my advisor, José Roberto da Cunha Lima, for all his guidance, patience, trust, encouragement and for motivating me to do this work, and especially for being such a professional.

To all the wonderful staff in the laboratories, Alexandra, Fabiana and Jordana, for their collaboration and support throughout the research. Thank you for everything.

Thank you very much to the people who consented to take part in the research, whose generosity made it possible to carry out the sensory acceptability stages.

"Almost anything is possible when you have dedication and skill. Great works are accomplished not by strength, but by perseverance."

(Samuel Johnson)

SUMMARY

Celiac disease (CD) is an autoimmune enteropathy caused by permanent gluten intolerance in genetically predisposed individuals, which causes damage to the mucosa of the small intestine, reducing the absorption of essential nutrients for the proper functioning of the body. It affects 0.3 to 1% of the world's population and around 0.89% of the Brazilian population. It is estimated that the prevalence of celiac disease affects around 300,000 people in Brazil. Of every eight people with the disease, only one is diagnosed. Currently, the only form of treatment for CD is the total and permanent removal of gluten from the diet. However, the greatest difficulty in feeding celiacs is access to products made with gluten-free ingredients that have sensory characteristics that are pleasing to the consumer. The gluten-free products available on the market are not produced on a large scale, are expensive and are inaccessible to the less economically favored social classes. The aim of this study was to produce gluten-free cookies from green banana flour as an alternative for people with celiac disease. This is an experimental study divided into: preparation development, physico-chemical analysis, acceptability test and statistical analysis of the data. The centesimal analysis showed that the percentage of moisture (52.743%), RMF (2.521%), lipids (30.362%), proteins (5.560%), carbohydrates (8.811%) and caloric value of the food was 330.752 Kcal/100g. In the acceptability test, the food was rated on appearance (83%), color (84%), taste (94%), texture (78%) and overall impression (89%). Therefore, the study proved to be a viable alternative for making food products from green banana flour, in order to expand the supply to people with CD, helping to promote quality of life.

Keywords: Celiac disease; Cookie; Green banana flour; Acceptability

1   INTRODUCTION

Celiac disease (CD) is currently a common condition in Brazil, as it is in other parts of the world. "It affects 0.3 to 1% of the world's population and around 0.89% of the Brazilian population (CATASSI; COBELLIS, 2007; FASANO; CATASSI, 2001). However, many cases remain undiagnosed for a long period of time (CROVELLA et al, 2007)." It is estimated that the prevalence of celiac disease affects around 2 million people in Brazil. Of every eight people with the disease, only one is diagnosed. This disease can occur at any stage of life, and currently one in 400 Brazilians may have the disease and not be diagnosed (FENACELBRA, 2013).

According to Pratesie et al. (2006), CD is considered a public health problem worldwide, mainly due to its high prevalence, frequent association with variable and non-specific morbidity and, in the long term, the increased likelihood of serious complications, especially osteoporosis and malignant diseases of the gastroenteric tract.

According to Moraes (2014), "CD is an autoimmune disease caused by permanent intolerance to gluten and causes damage to the mucosa of the small intestine, reducing the absorption of essential nutrients for the proper functioning of the body." Currently, the only treatment for CD is total and permanent withdrawal from gluten. However, "absolute restriction of gluten is a difficult task for sufferers of the disease (SDEPANIAN et al, 1999)." The importance of maintaining a strict diet lies in the fact that the disease not only causes digestive symptoms, but also anemia, skin lesions, osteopenia and adenocarcinoma of the small intestine (PEREIRA; FILHO, 2013).

However, the biggest difficulty in feeding celiacs is access to products made with gluten-free ingredients that have sensory characteristics that are pleasing to the consumer. The gluten-free products available on the market are not produced on a large scale, are expensive and become inaccessible to the less economically favored social classes.

Individuals with CD need gluten-free foods with sensory, nutritional and low-cost characteristics, in order to favor adherence to treatment and promote an increase in quality of life. In this sense, it is important to look for alternatives in order to develop other food options to expand the supply of products and provide greater acceptance of new eating patterns by people with CD.

This includes the use of bananas in gluten-free preparations. Bananas are the second most consumed fruit in the world, at 10.38 kg/inhab/year (FAO, 2011)." "Brazil is the 5th largest banana producer in the world." Banana growing is the 12$^\mathrm{a}$ most important crop in the country, ranking second in terms of the volume of fruit produced (FAO, 2014)." Banana consumption is growing every year due to the efforts of the production sector, which works to qualify production, and the marketing sector, which involves aspects of presentation as well as publicizing the benefits generated for the consumer. "The good acceptance of bananas is due to their pleasant sensory aspects, the absence of hard seeds and juice in the pulp, as well as their availability throughout the year (FASOLIN et al, 2007)."

The fruit is easily accessible to the population, low cost and high in nutritional properties. Found at all times of the year, "bananas are rich in minerals that are essential for the body, such as phosphorus, manganese, copper, iron, magnesium and calcium, as well as vitamins A, C and B complex (B1, B2 and niacin), in addition to pectin and resistant starch (FERREIRA et al, 2014)."

Resistant starch is a functional food and its action is similar to that of dietary fiber, as it is not digested in the small intestine. The undigested part that reaches the intestine acts as a prebiotic, being fermented by beneficial bacteria in the large intestine, producing short-chain fatty acids (SCFA), mainly butyrate, which prevent infections and intestinal cancer (MACHADO; SAMPAIO, 2013).

The use of resistant starch reduces the risk of cardiovascular disease, contributes to weight loss because it acts as a fiber, promoting a feeling of satiety for longer, reduces the risk of developing diabetes and helps in the treatment of diabetes mellitus, especially type 2 diabetes, by reducing the glycemic index of food. The best way to make use of resistant starch is to consume the banana while it is still green, making green banana flour, which has no taste and can be added to various preparations (FERREIRA et al, 2014).

Gluten is known to be present in cereals such as wheat, rye, barley, malt (a by-product of barley) and oats (BAPTISTA, 2006). In this sense, it is feasible to produce food using green banana flour as a substitute for gluten-containing ingredients, such as its use in the production of a nutritious gluten-free *cookie made from* green banana flour, as an alternative food among the options that already exist in the highly deprived market, which can meet the needs of celiacs, in order to meet the needs of those suffering from the disease.

In view of the above, the aim of this study was to produce gluten-free *cookies* made from green banana flour, since it is of great importance since green banana biomass has important nutritional characteristics. In addition, it represents yet another consumption option for an important part of the population that has restrictions on the consumption of gluten-containing products, with the aim of using it as an additional food for celiacs in order to promote a better quality of life.

2 OBJECTIVES

2.1 General

Research into *cookies* made from green banana flour as an alternative for people with celiac disease.

2.2 Specifics

- Demonstrate the nutritional properties of green bananas to produce green banana flour;

- Making a nutritious gluten-free *cookie* as an alternative for celiacs;

- To check the physico-chemical characteristics of *cookies* made from green banana flour;

- Carry out a sensory acceptability test of the *cookie*;

3 literary review

3.1 GLÛTEN

Gluten "is the main protein constituent of wheat, oats, rye and barley. In these cereals, the alcohol-soluble gluten fraction (called gliadin, avenin, hordein and secalin, respectively) is toxic to celiac patients (ACELBRA, 2016; NIEWINSKI, 2008)", which causes a chronic inflammatory state of the small intestinal mucosa accompanied by villous atrophy and hyperplasia of the intestinal crypts (LINDFORS, MAKI and KAUKINEN, 2010)." "This is because they are not completely hydrolyzed by human digestive enzymes in celiac patients (CRESPO, PÉREZ and CASTILLEJO, 2012)." This impairs the absorption of nutrients.

The use of gluten is fundamental in the production of bread, as it allows gases generated inside the molecules of cereals, particularly wheat, to be retained during biological fermentation, allowing the dough to expand and become softer (a phenomenon popularly known as bread growth). Without gluten, baking as we know it today would not be possible.

Gluten has technological properties that give products quality, such as elasticity and hydration, as well as helping to increase yields. Products without gluten have characteristics that are detrimental to quality, giving rise to products with small specific volumes, which are firmer and less durable (BOBBIO and BOBBIO, 2001).

However, it is necessary to develop and adapt alternative products, prepared for consumption by people with celiac disease, as well as to warn of the existence of gluten in conventional foods. Because of this, in order to guarantee the practice of a gluten-free diet, Federal Law number 8,543 (BRAZIL, 1992) was enacted in 1992, which requires the printing of the warning contains gluten on the labels and packaging of industrialized foods that contain derivatives of wheat, rye, barley and oats.

3.2 CELL DISEASE

Celiac disease (CD) "is an autoimmune disease triggered by the ingestion of cereals containing gluten, including barley, rye, wheat and malt (a by-product of barley), by genetically predisposed individuals (ARAÙJO et al, 2010)." "Studies show that CD usually manifests itself in childhood, between the first and third year of life, however, it can appear at any age, including adulthood (ACELBRA, 2009).

CD affects around 0.3 to 1% of the world's population and 0.89% of the Brazilian population (CATASSI; COBELLIS, 2007; FASANO; CATASSI, 2001). However, many cases remain undiagnosed for a long period of time (CROVELLA et al, 2007)." Thus, CD can be considered a public health problem worldwide, mainly due to its high prevalence, its frequent association with unspecified morbidity and, in the long term, the likelihood of serious complications, especially osteoporosis and malignant diseases of the gastrointestinal tract (PRATESI and GANDOLFI, 2006).

According to Sdepanian et al. (2001), the main manifestation of gluten intake in patients with celiac disease is the development of an inflammatory process that affects the mucosa of the small intestine in the duodeno-jejunal portion, triggering total or subtotal atrophy of the intestinal villi, with consequent difficulty in absorbing nutrients, among other symptoms.

According to Pereira and Filho (2013), CD can take four forms: classic, atypical, silent and latent. The classic form of CD is defined by symptoms and sequelae of gastrointestinal malabsorption. The diagnosis is established by serological tests and by the villous atrophy evident in the biopsy. Atypical CD, on the *other hand, is* characterized by few or no gastrointestinal symptoms, and extra intestinal manifestations are predominant. Atypical CD is the most common presentation today and is responsible for the increase in prevalence. Diagnosis is established in the same way as in classic CD. In silent CD, individuals are asymptomatic, but have a positive serological test and villous atrophy on biopsy. They are usually detected by selecting high-risk individuals or by performing an endoscopic duodenal biopsy. Latent CD is defined by positive serology, but without villous atrophy in the biopsy. These individuals are asymptomatic, but can later develop symptoms and histological changes.

The indication of a lifelong gluten-free diet for CD sufferers is an international consensus, although in the so-called asymptomatic forms it is still highly questioned. As the histological changes in the small intestine may be the same as in those with symptoms, it is assumed that even asymptomatic individuals are at risk in the long term and should be placed on a gluten-free diet. Patients with the silent form or with mild symptoms are possibly at greater risk of health problems, due to the difficulty of diagnosis and the delay in introducing treatment (BAPTISTA, 2006).

3.3 GLUTEN-FREE DIET

Strict adherence to a gluten-free diet throughout life is of fundamental importance in order to eliminate symptoms and restore the normal morphology of the intestinal mucosa, to ensure proper development, reduce the risk of macro- and micronutrient deficiencies, and consequently reduce the risk of malignant diseases, particularly of the digestive system. Starting treatment with a gluten-free diet quickly reverses mucosal damage and corrects malabsorption with a significant improvement in symptoms (SIQUEIRA NETO et al, 2004; LEFFLER et al, 2009).

Although most patients who follow a gluten-free diet comply with the restricted diet, it is problematic in terms of cost and nutritional value (LEFFLER et al, 2009). Symptom improvement is usually seen within days of starting the gluten-free diet, while complete mucosal recovery usually takes longer (BRIANI; SAMARO; ALAEDINI, 2008).

Although the absence of gluten from diets provides a significant improvement in symptoms, the nutritional quality of the food produced is not guaranteed. Technological advances have led to the development of foods that are pleasant for celiacs (KOHMANN, 2010). However, gluten-free products are generally made with refined flours and starches, and therefore have a low content of dietary fiber, vitamins and minerals, which is one of the factors responsible for the inadequate consumption of these nutrients by celiacs (THONPSOM et al., 2005).

However, adhering to a completely gluten-free diet is not an easy practice due to the difficulty of adapting to modified products, cross-contamination with cereals containing gluten, inadequate labeling and the lack of gluten-free products on the market (ZANDONADI, 2009). The trade in foods for celiacs is still limited and the cost of those sold is high, making it essential to develop new food products for this population. In response to this need, research has emerged to make it possible to use gluten-free raw materials with added nutritional value to make new foods.

3.4 BANANA

3.5 BOTANICAL CLASSIFICATION OF BANANAS

According to the nomenclature created by Linneo in 1735 (MINHOTO, 2006), bananas belong to the genus Musa, within the class *Monocotyledoneae,* order *Scimitales,* family *Musaceae and* subfamily *Musoideae,* which has two genera: the genus *Musa,* where the edible and technologically interesting fruits are found, is represented by around 30 species and the genus *Ensete* with ornamental fruits.

Currently, the classification system adopted for edible banana plants is based on the work of Simmonds and Shepherd (1955), who used a scoring method to indicate the relative contributions of two wild species (*M.* acuminata and *M.* balbisiana) in the genetic makeup of a given cultivar (VILAS BOAS *et al.,* 2001). The combination of these genomes results in the genomic groups: diploids AA, BB, AB; triploids AAA, AAB, ABB and tetraploids AAAA, AAAB, AABB, ABBB, this classification being adopted worldwide (DANTAS; SOARES FILHO, 1997).

In addition to the genomic groups, the term subgroup was used to refer to a complex of cultivars that originated through mutations of a single original cultivar, as in the case of the AAA group, the Cavendish subgroup, and the AAB group, the Prata and Terra subgroups, in Brazil.

3.5.1 Variety

According to EMBRAPA (2009), the most widespread varieties in Brazil are Prata, Pacovan, Prata Anâ, Maça, Mysore, Terra and D'Angola, from the AAB group, used solely for the domestic market, and Nanica, Nanicao and Grande Naine, from the AAA group, used mainly for export. On a smaller scale, Ouro (AA), Fingo Cinza and

Figo Vermelho (ABB), Caru Verde and Caru Roxa (AAA) are planted. The Prata, Prata Anâ and Pacovan varieties account for approximately 60% of the area under banana cultivation in Brazil.

3.5.2 NUTRITIONAL COMPOSITION OF GREEN BANANAS

The banana, regardless of its genomic group, is undoubtedly one of the most consumed fruits in the world. It is a highly energetic food (around 100 kcal per 100 g of pulp), whose carbohydrates, around 22%, are easily assimilated. Although low in protein and lipids, its content exceeds that of apples, pears, cherries and peaches. It contains as much vitamin C as apples, as well as reasonable amounts of vitamin A B1, B2, small amounts of vitamins D and E, and a higher percentage of potassium, phosphorus, calcium and iron than apples or oranges (EMBRAPA, 1997).

In green bananas (BV), the main component is starch, which can account for 55 to 93% of the total solids content. In ripe bananas, the starch is converted into sugars, mostly glucose, fructose and sucrose, 99.5% of which is physiologically available. Depending on the cultivar, the fruit can weigh from 100 to 200 grams or more, containing 60 to 65% edible pulp (MEDINA, 1995).

According to Giacobbo (2013), the diet enriched with green banana has been the subject of some research in Brazil due to its nutritional properties and especially due to its high content of insoluble and non-digestible fiber, characteristics that give this product the potential to be used as a parebiotic, in other words, a non-digestible food that has a beneficial effect on the body, revealing significant benefits for some ailments such as colorectal cancer, diarrhea, glycemic index, insulin response, dyslipidemia, cardiovascular disease and celiac disease, the latter of which was discussed by Zandonadi (2009).

3.6 RESISTANT STARCH FROM GREEN BANANAS

Among the main components of green bananas is resistant starch (RS), which can account for 55 to 93% of the total solids content, and fibers around 14.5% (OVANDO-MARTINEZ, 2009). When bananas ripen, resistant starch is converted into sugars, mostly glucose, fructose and sucrose, 99.5% of which are physiologically available (FASOLIN et al, 2007).

According to (PEREIRA, 2007), clinical studies have shown that resistant starch has properties similar to dietary fiber, acting as a functional food and showing physiological benefits in humans, and may act in the prevention of diseases. However, in relation to soluble dietary fibers, which are rapidly fermented by bacteria in the large intestine to produce Short Chain Fatty Acids (SCFA), such as acetate, propionate and especially butyrate, which act on colon health. RA has the benefit of not causing gastrointestinal discomfort, as it is fermented more slowly and therefore does not lead to the production of gas. The slow digestion of RA can improve the glycemic and insulinemic response with a relevant effect on the control of metabolic syndrome, which is responsible for some of the biggest health problems today: obesity, cardiovascular diseases and diabetes (VAN DOKKUM, 2008).

The functional properties of starch isolated from green banana pulp and flour from green fruit pulp were studied by Lobo and Lemos (2003), who found that dried, finely ground pulp has properties similar to those of isolated starch, thus raising the possibility of using bananas *in the* form of flour, which would allow the use of fruit rejected for sale *in natura*.

According to Zhang et al. (2005), green banana starch has great potential. In addition to its digestive and functional properties, it has applications in food processing, which makes its production commercially viable.

Resistant starch can be classified into four types: AR1, AR2, AR3 and AR4. The ARI type is physically inaccessible, as it is present in grains and seeds that are partially crushable due to the presence of rigid cell walls. Type AR2 is found in raw potatoes and green bananas. AR3 arises from the process of starch retrogradation, which is very common in processed, cooked and chilled foods. The AR4 type consists of chemically modified starch (SALGADO, 2005).

The presence of starch in the preparation of products is of interest to both the food industry and the consumer. Starch can be used in the preparation of products with a low lipid or sugar content and helps to increase the volume of products by absorbing water (LAJOLO et al., 2001). It also has physiological functions such as intestinal regulation, glycemic control, delayed gastric emptying and can help control cholesterol (LANGKILDE et al., 2002).

3.7 FUNCTIONAL FOODS

The term "functional food" was first used in Japan for food products that, in addition to nutritional functions, had some positive impact on special physiological functions (SIRÓ et al., 2008). the risk of becoming ill. Generally speaking, functional foods are defined as substances or components of a food that are capable of providing health benefits not obtained from the consumption of a single conventional food (BERNARDES et al., 2010).

Functional foods are those that come from the opportunity to combine highly flexible edible products with biologically active molecules, as a strategy to improve metabolic disorders, resulting in reduced risk of disease and health maintenance, in addition to the nutritional value inherent in their chemical composition (BERNARDES et al., 2010).

A food can be considered functional if it is demonstrated that it can beneficially affect one or more target functions in the body, in addition to possessing the appropriate nutritional effects, in a way that is both relevant to well-being and health and to reducing the risk of a disease (ROBERFROID, 2002). Functional foods are foods that provide the opportunity to combine highly flexible edible products with biologically active molecules, as a strategy to consistently correct metabolic disorders (WALZEM, 2004), resulting in reduced risk of disease and health maintenance (ANJO, 2004).

Functional foods are characterized by offering various health benefits, in addition to the nutritional value inherent in their chemical composition, and can potentially play a beneficial role in reducing the risk of chronic degenerative diseases (NEUMANN, et al., 2002; TAIPINA, et al., 2002).

According to (SOUZA, et al., 2003), functional foods and ingredients can be classified in two ways: in terms of their source, whether of plant or animal origin, or in terms of the benefits they offer, acting in six areas of the body: in the gastrointestinal system; in the cardiovascular system; in the metabolism of substrates; in growth, development and cell differentiation; in the behavior of physiological functions and as antioxidants.

Kruger & Mann (2003) define functional ingredients as a group of compounds that have health benefits, such as allicins found in garlic, carotenoids and flavonoids found in fruit and vegetables, glucosinolates found in cruciferous vegetables, polyunsaturated fatty acids found in vegetable oils and fish oil. These ingredients can be consumed together with the foods from which they come, and these foods are considered functional foods.

3.8 GREEN BANANA FLOUR AND ITS POTENTIAL CULINARY USE

The pulp of green bananas, which can be dehydrated, contains 70 to 80 % starch, an amount that can be compared to the endosperm of grains such as corn and vegetables such as potatoes (ZHANG et al., 2005).

The literature highlights the use of green banana pulp in food production, as it does not alter the taste, increases the amount of fiber, proteins and minerals, and increases the yield of preparations due to water absorption (VALLE; CAMARGOS, 2003).

Bananas have around 100 kcal per 100g of pulp and, although they are low in protein and lipids, their content exceeds that of other fruits such as apples, pears and peaches. They contain as much vitamin C as apples, as well as reasonable amounts of vitamin A, B1, B2, small amounts of vitamin D and E, and a higher percentage of potassium, phosphorus and calcium than apples and oranges (FASOLIN et al., 2007).

By dehydrating the green banana pulp, it is possible to obtain green banana flour, which has a mild flavor and can replace other flours without damaging the sensory characteristics (LOBO; SILVA, 2003). Green banana flour can be used as a nutritional enhancement for soups, porridges, pancake batters, soufflés, pizzas and other products (FASOLIN et al., 2007).

According to Zandonadi (2009), the use of green banana flour in food production, as well as being a possibility for the development of special-purpose foods for celiac patients, stands out as an alternative for minimizing the production of solid waste, with a consequent reduction in waste in the marketing of bananas, as well as presenting the possibility of a nutritional increase. These factors stand out in terms of helping to prevent diseases and improving quality of life.

3.9 CORN STARCH

Cornstarch is a dry, powdery carbohydrate with no special flavor. The use of starch gives preparations a gelatinous and delicate consistency. Extracted from corn kernels. It is gluten-free and has no taste or smell. It is a fine, smooth, white powder (ACELPAR, 2010).

Corn starch plays a structural role in pasta and bread. During baking, the starch granules absorb water, swell and stiffen, and the process of gelatinization takes place. Starch can be used as a thickener in sauces, soups, puddings and in the production of cakes and cookies, promoting a fine, compact texture. Like starch, other corn derivatives, such as flour and cornmeal, in association with other ingredients that are a source of fat (oils, margarine, butter), can be used in gluten-free preparations such as cakes and cookies (ATZINGEN; PINTO-E-SILVA, 2005).

3.10 BISCUITS

A cookie or cracker is a product obtained by kneading and baking dough prepared with flours, starches, fermented or unfermented starches and other food substances (SIMBESP, 2016).

Among bakery products, cookies are of great commercial interest due to their production, consumption, shelf-life and acceptance characteristics. Many of these products have been created with the aim of improving their nutritional formulation (CATASSI; FASANO, 2008; PEREZ; GERMANI, 2007).

Brazil is the world's fourth largest cookie producer, with 1.2 million tons/year in 2015, surpassed only by China (3.4 million tons), the United States (2.3 million tons) and India (1.9 million tons). Per capita consumption in 2015 was 6.0 kg/year, making it fifth in the world. On the national scene, it is a market that generated more than 21 billion reais in 2015, representing an increase of more than 48% compared to 2011, when it generated just over 14 billion, demonstrating the growth of this product over the years (ABIMAPI, 2016).

Although they are not a staple food like bread, cookies are accepted and consumed by people of all ages. Their long shelf life allows them to be produced in large quantities and widely distributed. A product with such characteristics, combined with its enormous diversity, presents itself as a good vehicle for the study of mixed flours, whether for economic or nutritional reasons (EL-DASH; GERMANI, 1994).

3.10.1 Sensory characteristics of cookies

Cookies must have the appearance of toasted dough, their own color, smell and taste (MORRETO; FETT, 1999). It is therefore necessary to know the most important sensory attributes for this product, knowing that sensory quality is the main factor in the acceptance and preference of cookies.

The consumer's first contact with a product is usually with its visual presentation, where color and appearance stand out. Every product has an expected appearance and color that are associated with personal reactions of acceptance, indifference or rejection. The form is usually related to the natural form, or to a culturally established commercial form (TEIXEIRA, 2009).

According to Lermen et al. (2015), in order for an unknown product to be consumed, it needs to attract the consumer, but it is essential that the product has a good appearance in order to be consumed, so it needs to have a good appearance, slightly shiny, without the appearance of overcooked or lightly cooked dough.

According to Lermen et al. (2015), odor is one of the characteristics of a product that has the capacity to attract or repel consumers, and is of great importance in the acceptance of food products. Odor can indicate to the consumer the quality and healthiness of the product.

Taste is one of the sensory properties of the oral cavity related to taste, perceived in the mouth (TEIXEIRA, 2009). Taste is a complex attribute, defined as a mixed but unitary experience of olfactory, gustatory and tactile sensations perceived during tasting (LERMEN et al., 2015).

According to Lermen et al. (2015), smell and taste are related and it is only possible to taste food through the two senses of smell and taste. Taste receptors are activated by substances present in food and olfactory receptors are activated by substances present in the air, but much of what people call taste is the result of smell, because when certain foods are broken down during chewing, the smell spreads through the nose.

The odor and taste characteristics of the product must be designed to appeal to the target audience, since its acceptance will depend on the taste and psychological characteristics of the consumer, and there must be a balance between the taste and odor of the products (LERMEN et al., 2015).

Since consumer satisfaction comes from their positive perception of the quality of the food, it should be borne in mind that it is the consumer themselves who should dictate the quality parameters of this product. In studies involving the sensory analysis of food, such as those focused on acceptance and preference tests, the consumer is the fundamental object of measuring the sensory quality of the product. There is no point in a food having desirable physical, chemical and microbiological qualities, or being superior to its competitors, if it does not have the backing of the consumer in terms of its appearance, aroma, taste and texture (DELA LUCIA, 2008).

3.10.2 Gluten-free cookies

According to Zucco et al. (2011), it is possible to find gluten-free cookies on the market, but many of the products available are not well accepted by consumers. In addition, they have little nutritional value and a high cost, making them difficult to access for economically disadvantaged populations (RODRIGUES FERREIRA et al., 2009).

In the preparation of gluten-free cookies and bakery products, rice flour, rice cream, corn starch, sweet potato flour, cornmeal, cassava flour, sweet starch, sour starch and potato starch are some of the options of ingredients that can be used (CÉSAR et al., 2006).

Various studies have evaluated the replacement of wheat flour with gluten-free flours, with the aim of offering consumers differentiated products from a technological and nutritional point of view, especially products such as cookies, bread and cakes, among others. In this sense, green banana biomass can be used in gluten-free preparations, especially in the development of bakery products such as cookies.

3.11 LEGISLATION ON FOOD LABELING

To ensure a gluten-free diet, "celiacs should always know the ingredients that make up food preparations and read the ingredients listed on the labels of industrialized products (ARAÙJO et al, 2010)." Paying attention to the inscriptions "does not contain gluten" or "contains gluten", as a measure to control celiac disease (BRASIL, 2003). This measure makes it easier and gives celiac patients more confidence when choosing foods for their diet.

In 2002, the National Health Surveillance Agency (ANVISA) created RDC No. 40, of February 8, 2002, published in the Official Gazette of February 13, 2002, which approves the Technical Regulations for labeling packaged foods and beverages containing gluten. All packaged foods and beverages containing gluten, such as wheat, oats, barley, malt (a by-product of barley) and rye, must contain the warning on the label: "contains gluten". The warning must be printed on the labels of packaged foods and drinks in clear, easily readable characters (ANVISA, 2002). In May 2003, Federal Law No. 10674 was created, amending RDC No. 40 of 2002. Under Federal Law No. 10.674, food products that are marketed must be informed of the presence of gluten, as a preventative measure and to control celiac disease, and all industrialized foods must be labelled with the words "contains gluten" or "does not contain gluten", as appropriate (ANVISA, 2003).

However, it remains to be defined as law that warnings about the presence of gluten must be placed on ready meals served in restaurants that offer meals by weight, and on their display menus. Awareness in the food sector must be raised in order to include celiacs and guarantee food that is free from cross-contamination.

4 METHODOLOGY

The methodology was used to clarify how the research was carried out in order to develop gluten-free cookies from green banana flour as an alternative for people with celiac disease. This study was based on bibliographical research, reading various theoretical sources and exploratory research in order to understand fundamental information about the importance of the nutritional properties of green banana biomass and its use in the production of cookies as an alternative for people with celiac disease.

4.1 CHARACTERIZATION OF THE TYPE OF STUDY AND APPROACH

This study was characterized as descriptive, exploratory, field and bibliographic research, with a quantitative and qualitative approach. According to Cesino (2010), scientific research is descriptive when it is carried out through surveys or systematic observations of known characteristics, components of the fact/process, seeking to describe a reality without interfering in it. The researcher simply records and describes the facts observed without interfering in them, seeking to discover the frequency with which a fact occurs, its nature, its characteristics, causes and its relationship with other facts (PRODANOV and FREITAS, 2013).

The exploratory type, because the research is in the preliminary phase, aims to provide more information on the subject to be investigated, making it possible to define and outline it, facilitating the delimitation of the research topic and guiding the setting of objectives and the formulation of hypotheses or discovering a new type of approach to the subject (PRODANOV and FREITAS, 2013).

The procedure used in the work was fieldwork, which according to PRODANOV and FREITAS (2013), "is used with the aim of obtaining information and knowledge about a problem for which an answer is sought." It consists of observing facts and collecting data relating to the research and recording variables that we assume to be relevant, in order to analyze them (PRODANOV and FREITAS, 2013). It was of the bibliographical type, as we used already published materials, consisting mainly of books, magazines and scientific articles, with the aim of putting the researcher in direct contact with all the material already written on the subject of the research (PRODANOV and FREITAS, 2013). The approach was quantitative "because it can be quantified, which means translating opinions and information into numbers in order to classify and analyze them (PRODANOV and FREITAS, 2013)". It is qualitative because it considers that there is a dynamic relationship between the real world and the subject, that is, an inseparable link between the objective world and the subject's subjectivity that cannot be translated into numbers.

It does not require the use of statistical methods and techniques. The natural environment is the direct source of data collection and the researcher is the key instrument (PRODANOV; FREITAS, 2013).

4.2 METHODOLOGICAL PROCEDURES

The *cookie* cookies made in this study had their recipes adapted from cooking websites and books. Factors such as practicality of preparation and sensory aspects such as color, aroma, texture and taste were taken into account when selecting the recipes.

The preparations were made in the Technique and Dietetics Laboratory and the physico-chemical analyses were carried out in the Chemistry and Bromatology Laboratory of the Mauricio de Nassau College (FMN) - FAP Parnaiba Unit and all the costs of preparing the work were the responsibility of the academic. During the preparation of the recipes, the data relating to the preparation was recorded, such as: weight of the ingredients used in grams and in homemade measures, gross weight, net weight, ingredient correction factor and weight of the finished preparations. This data is necessary for the preparation of the technical sheets of the preparations and for checking the nutrients. DIGIPESO DP-03 digital scales were used to weigh the food[®].

4.3 POPULATION AND SAMPLE

The research into the acceptability of the green banana flour *cookie* was carried out in a supermarket in the city of Parnaiba with customers of both sexes, aged between 16 and 63, in a total of 50 people.

The study sample was composed by convenience (voluntary sampling), in which the researcher invited clients individually to take part in the research. Those who agreed to be part of the sample signed an Informed Consent Form (ICF) and evaluated the preparation according to the acceptability questionnaire.

4.4 PREPARATION OF FORMULATIONS

4.4.1 RAW MATERIALS

The formulations shown in Table 1 were used to make the *cookie,* using the following ingredients: Green banana flour made in the Technique and Dietetics laboratory of the Mauricio de Nassau College - FAP unit, Parnaiba, brown sugar, corn starch, unsalted butter, sodium bicarbonate, salt, whole chicken eggs, vanilla flavoring and Brazil nuts. All the products used were sourced from suppliers in the region where the cookies were made.

4.5 MAKING GREEN BANANA FLOUR

The raw materials were weighed on a DIGIPESO DP-03 ® digital scale, then dropped and sanitized under running water. They were then immersed in chlorine solution (200 ppm) for 15 minutes. The green bananas were then placed in a pressure cooker with the peel on and the water was added halfway up. Cover the pot and wait until steam starts coming out of the valve, then leave to cook for 10 minutes. After this time, turn off the heat and wait until the pan naturally loses pressure. Then the pan was uncovered, the cooked bananas were cut into slices of approximately 1 cm using a knife, and placed on a baking sheet in the oven at 200 °C to dry completely. Then they were taken out of the oven and left to cool at room temperature, after which the dehydrated banana slices were ground in a blender until flour was obtained.

4.6 DEVELOPMENT OF *COOKIES*

The ingredients were first weighed individually on a DIGIPESO DP-03 digital scale[®]
. After weighing, the ingredients were

mixed in an ARNO domestic mixer[®] . The butter and sugar were added and mixed for about 3 minutes, obtaining an aerated mixture, then the egg, green banana flour, cornstarch were added and mixed until homogeneous, and finally the salt and baking soda were added, mixed for 5 minutes until a dough was obtained, then the mixer was turned off and the dough was mixed with the Brazil nuts. Once the dough was ready, it was left to rest in the fridge for 30 minutes. The dough was then shaped by hand and placed on a greased baking tray, then placed in a SUGGAR electric oven[®] , with capacity for two mats and temperature control, where the cookies were baked for 15 minutes at a temperature of 180 °C. After baking, the cookies were cooled to room temperature and placed in containers.

TABLE 1: Ingredients used in the formulation of *cookies made* from green banana flour.

INGREDIENTS	QUANTITY (g)	HOMEMADE MEASURE
Green banana flour	110	¾ cup
Corn starch	58	½ cup
Brown sugar	100	½ cup
Butter	50	2 full tablespoons
Sodium bicarbonate	3	1 teaspoon
Vanilla essence	10	1 tablespoon
Egg	50	1 unit
Brazil nuts	50	½ cup
Salt	I	1 level teaspoon

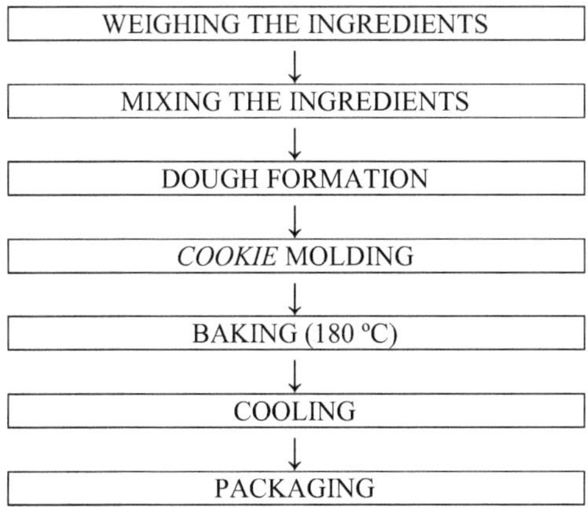

Figure 1: Biscuit preparation flowchart

4.7 PHYSICAL AND CHEMICAL CHARACTERIZATION

Determinations of pH, moisture, protein, ash and lipids were carried out in triplicate according to INSTITUTO ADOLFO LUTZ (IAL, 2008).

4.8 pH DETERMINATION

To determine PH, 10 g of the sample was weighed into a beaker and diluted with 100 mL of water. The contents were stirred with a stirrer for 10 minutes until the particles, if any, were evenly suspended and left to rest for six minutes. The pH was then determined using the previously calibrated apparatus, operating it according to the instructions in the manufacturer's manual, taking three readings on the sample.

4.9 HUMIDITY

Three crucibles were weighed individually on the BIOPRECISA® analytical balance and the weight noted. Then 5 g of the *cookie* sample was weighed into each crucible and the weight noted. The cookie was placed in a FANEM® oven at 105° C (check that the oven thermometer was reading this temperature) and allowed to dry for one hour. Once this time had elapsed, the samples were placed in a desiccator and waited 15 minutes for them to cool down in order to avoid variations during weighing. Finally, the crucible with the dry sample after cooling was weighed.

Calculation:

$$\% \text{ humidity at } 105\ ^\circ C\ p/p\ \square\ \frac{100*N}{P}$$

N: weight loss in grams

P: gram mass of the sample

4.10 TOTAL MINERALS (ash)

Three crucibles were weighed individually on the BIOPRECISA® analytical balance and the weight noted. Then 2 g of the *cookie* sample was weighed into each crucible and the weight noted. The samples were placed in a muffle furnace previously heated to 550°C for incineration until the ashes turned white or slightly gray. They were then cooled in a desiccator to room temperature and weighed again. The heating and cooling operations were repeated until constant weight.

Calculation:

$$\% \text{ Ash at } 550\ °C\ p/p = \frac{100*N}{P}$$

N = number of grams of ash

P = number of grams of sample

4.11 PROTEINS

To start the digestion or mineralization, a 0.25 sample was weighed on an analytical balance according to the procedure and 2.5g of the catalytic mixture and 7mL of sulphuric acid P.A. were added. The digestion block was heated slowly at first, keeping the temperature at $50°$ C for an hour. The temperature was then gradually raised to $400°$ C until the liquid became clear and transparent, with a blue-green tint. It was removed from the heat and allowed to cool, after which 10 mL of water was added.

For the distillation, the Erlenmeyer flask containing 20 mL of 4% boric acid with 4 to 5 drops of mixed indicator solution was attached to the distiller. The Kjeldahl tube was fitted to the distiller and the 50% sodium hydroxide solution was added until it turned black (about 20 mL). Distillation was carried out, testing with pH indicator paper until no more alkaline reaction occurred. The receiving solution was kept cold during distillation. It was titrated with 0.1N sulfuric acid solution or 0.1N hydrochloric acid solution until the indicator turned.

Calculations:

$$\% \text{ total nitrogen} = \frac{V*N*f*0.014*100}{P}$$

$$\% \text{ protein} = \% \text{ total nitrogen} * F$$

Where:

V: milliliters of 0.1 N sulfuric acid solution or 0.1 N hydrochloric acid solution used in the titration, after correction of the blank

N: theoretical normality of 0.1N sulfuric acid solution or 0.1N hydrochloric acid solution

f: correction factor of 0.1N sulfuric acid solution or 0.1N hydrochloric acid solution

P: sample mass in grams

F: nitrogen/protein ratio conversion factor, according to the product

The weighed and dried Soxhlet cartridge was weighed. Weigh 2 g of the sample into the Soxhlet cartridge. The cartridge was transferred to the Soxhlet extractor. Sufficient chloroform was added for one and a half Soxhlets. It was kept under continuous heating. The cartridge with the extracted residue was removed and placed in an oven at 105°C for about an hour. It was cooled in a desiccator to room temperature. It was then weighed and the heating operations repeated for 30 minutes in the oven and cooled to constant weight (maximum 2 hours).

Calculation:

$\dfrac{100 \times N}{P}$ = lipids or stereo extract percent m/m

N = number of grams of lipid = [(Cartridge weight + sample) - Final weight]

P = number of grams of sample

4.13 TOTAL CARBOHYDRATES

The glycemic fraction is determined by subtracting the sum of the nutrients from 100. The fiber portion of the food can be included in the glycemic fraction. When fiber is determined separately, this result is included in the sum of the nutrients.

Calculation:

GLYCIDIOS = 100 - (% moisture + % RMF + % proteins + % lipids)

Conversion factors were used, according to the methodology of Osborne and Voogt (1978), considering 4 kcal/g for proteins, 4 kcal/g for carbohydrates and 9 kcal/g for lipids. The result was expressed in kcal/100 g, based on the equation:

VC = (% protein x 4) + (% lipids x 9) + (% carbohydrates x 4).

1.15 CHECKING THE ACCEPTABILITY OF THE PREPARATION

The acceptability test was carried out with 50 (fifty) participants who were invited by the academic responsible for the research at random from among the customers who were in a supermarket in the city of Parnaiba - Piaui, where the importance of the test was explained.

To check the degree of acceptability of the *cookie*, an acceptability questionnaire was used with a nine-point structured hedonic scale ranging from very much liked (maximum score) to disliked (maximum score).

I liked it very much (minimum score), where the following items were added: age, gender, name of the preparation and comments. The questionnaire was used to evaluate the taste, appearance, texture, color and overall impression of the *cookie,* with each participant receiving a questionnaire to evaluate the preparation, as specified in Appendix A.

1.16 ACCEPTABILITY INDEX

The Acceptability Index (A.I.) of the product was calculated for each attribute evaluated in the sensory analysis as presented by Cunha et al (2010) following the equation, which has been used by numerous authors to express the acceptability of a product as a whole.

Calculation:

1. A (%) = (A x 100)

B

Where (A) represents the average of the attribute and (B) the highest score observed in the evaluated attribute.

1.17 ETHICAL AND LEGAL ASPECTS

This research followed ethical procedures, in which the participants signed the Informed Consent Form (ICF) and were informed about the objectives of the study and data collection. Those who agreed to take part in the research signed the ICF in two copies and kept one copy in their possession, the other being sent to the academic along with the questionnaire.

1.18 STATISTICAL ANALYSIS

The analysis and tabulation of the data obtained at the end of the study was carried out using Microsoft Excel 2010 spreadsheets. Subsequently, evaluations were made using descriptive statistics, mean and standard deviation.

5 Results and discussion

5.1 PHYSICAL AND CHEMICAL CHARACTERIZATION

The results obtained from the analysis of the cookie's centesimal composition are shown in Table 2 for each analysis, accompanied by the mean and standard deviation values.

ANALYSIS CENTESIMAL	AMOSTKA I	AMOSTKA II	AMOSTKA III	MEDLA	DEVIATION P.ADKÀO	CALORIC VALUE
HUMIDITY	53,488	53,678	51,063	52,743	1,457	0,000
RMF	2,523	2,569	2,470	2,521	0,049	0,000
ETHERIC EXTRACT	32,213	28,518	30,355	30,362	2,612	273,263 Kcal
PROTEINS	4,691	5,680	6,310	5,560	0,699	22,241 Kcal
CARBOHYDRATES	7,082	9,553	9,799	8,811	1,746	35,247 Kcal
pH	8,160	8,180	8,170	8,170	0,010	330,752 Kcal

TABLE2: Results of the cookie's centesimal analysis.

The physicochemical analysis showed that the cookie had a high moisture content, possibly due to the high amount of fiber in the green banana, which contributes to the retention of liquids.

According to Silva (2010), the moisture content of a food is related to its stability, quality and composition, and can directly affect its storage, processing and packaging. As cookies have a relatively low moisture content, they generally have a long shelf life. With regard to the limits established in legislation, it should be noted that CNNPA Resolution No. 12 of 1978, of the National Commission of Norms and Standards for Food (BRAZIL, 1978), which established a maximum moisture content of 14% for cookies and crackers, was revoked by RDC Resolution No. 263, of September 22, 2005, by ANVISA - Agência Nacional de Vigilância Sanitaria (BRAZIL, 2005), which approved the Technical Regulation for Cereal Products, Starches, Flours and Bran, however, it does not set limits for the moisture content of cookies.

The lipid values found are highly altered, possibly due to the vegetable fat added in the preparation, the use of a greased pan and the addition of Brazil nuts, which contain a significant amount of lipids. This value is higher when compared to the labels of commercially available cookies, which show average values ranging from 14% to 23% (REINERI and VALENTE, 2013). With regard to the ash content, the levels of mineral residue were in line with the recommended parameters, conforming to the values established by the Brazilian legislation ANVISA (BRASIL, 2001), which establishes levels of up to 3.0% mineral residue. The pH value for cookies is in the range close to normal for this product, generally between 6.5 and 8, as PYLER (1982) pointed out. LIMA (1988) found similar values for crackers (7.10). MENDONZA et al, (2004) evaluated commercial crackers and found similar pH values. The cookie produced had a calorific value of 330.752 Kcal/100g of the product, lower than that found by Perez and Germani (2007) who found 432.53 kcal.100 g-1 of cookies made with eggplant flour as a substitute for whole wheat flour, a lower percentage than the amount of FBV used in the cookie produced using 60% green banana, but a higher energy value. Rodrigues et al. (2007) made 3 types of cookies containing coffee and obtained caloric values of between 498 and 502 kcal.100 g-1 of the product, which were also higher than those found in this study.

5.2 CHECKING THE ACCEPTABILITY OF PREPARATIONS

The acceptability of the cookies was assessed using a 9-point structured hedonic scale, with scores ranging from strongly dislike (1) to strongly like (9) (DUTCOSKY, 2007). The analysis was carried out with 50 participants who agreed to take part in the survey. Table 2 shows that the majority of the individuals who took part in the study were female (62%) and with regard to age, it can be seen that the largest proportion was between 16 and 25 years old. The data obtained through the acceptability test was statistically able to raise averages for overall impression of the product, texture, color, appearance and taste.

TABLE 3: Socio-demographic characteristics of the participants

PARTICIPANTS		
SEX	N^0	%
F	31	62
M	19	38

ETARLA RANGE	N^0	%
16-25	17	34
26-35	9	18
36-45	10	20
46-55	7	14
56-65	7	14

After answering the above questions, the participants answered questions related to sensory attributes, looking at global aspects of the cookie and specific sensory parameters such as texture, color, appearance and taste.

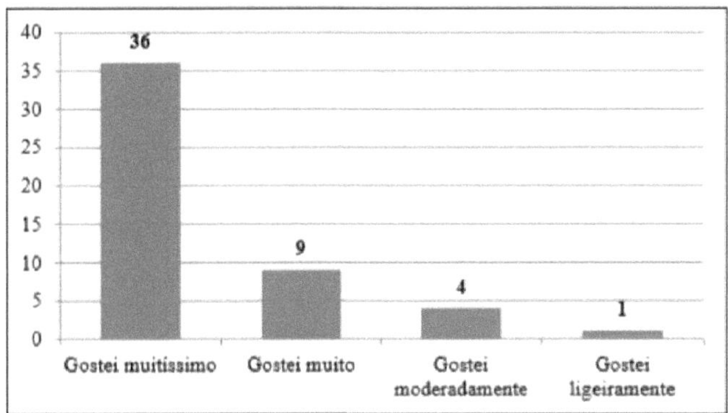

GRAPH 1: Number of nominations per item for the appearance attribute of the cookie made from green banana flour (Source: Research data).

As for the appearance attribute, (graph 1) shows that the majority (36) of the evaluators gave this attribute a score of 9. The other scores were as follows: I liked it very much, score 8 (09), I liked it moderately, score 7 (04) and I liked it a little (01).

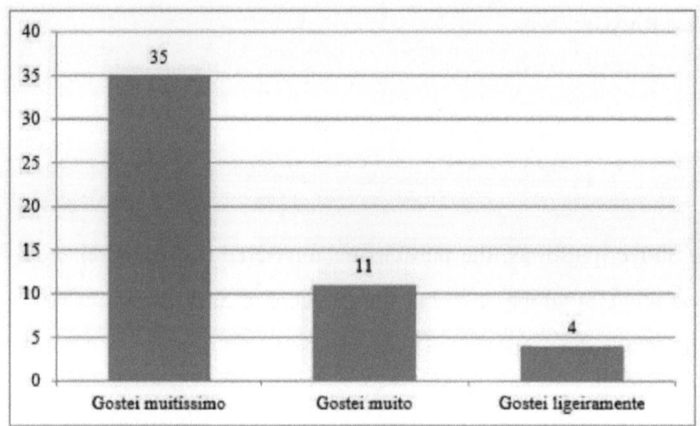

GRAPH 2: Number of indications per item for the color attribute of the cookie made from green banana flour (Source: Research data).

When evaluating the color attribute (Graph 2), it was found that the majority (35) of the tasters gave a score of 9 according to the hedonic scale, score 8 (11) and score 6 (04).

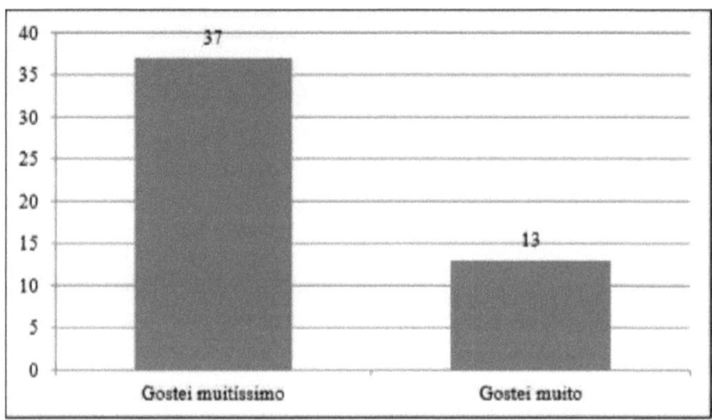

GRAPH 3: Number of nominations per item for the taste attribute of the cookie made from green banana flour (Source: Research data).

With regard to the taste attribute (Graph 3), the majority (37) gave a score of 9, which means I liked it very much according to the hedonic scale. The majority (37) gave a score of 9, which means I liked it very much, according to the hedonic scale, and the majority (13) gave a score of 8. No scores were given for scores of 7, 6, 5, 4, 3, 2 and 1.

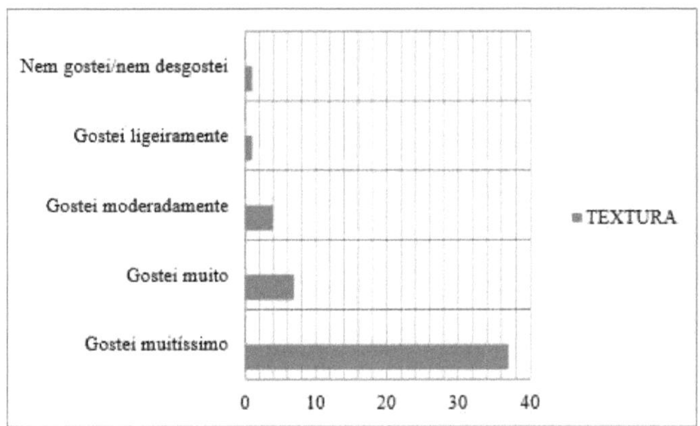

GRAPH 4: Number of nominations per item for the texture attribute of the cookie made from green banana flour (Source: Research data).

With regard to the texture attribute (Graph 4), the majority of tasters gave scores of 9, 8 and 7, so I liked it very much (37), I liked it a lot (07) and I liked it moderately (04), while I liked it slightly and neither liked it nor disliked it scored 6 on the hedonic scale with (01) score each.

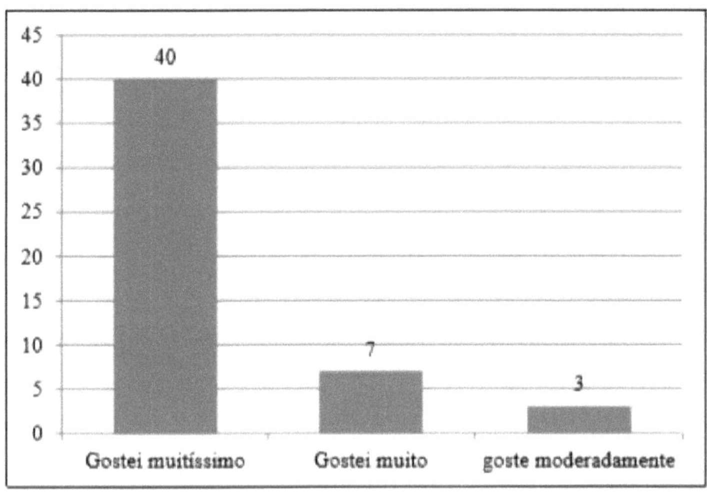

GRAPH 5: Number of nominations per item for the overall impression attribute of the cookie made from green banana flour (Source: Research data).

The overall impression was an attribute that was well accepted by the tasters. The majority (40) gave it a score of 9, i.e. I liked it very much, according to the hedonic scale. The overall impression expresses how much the evaluator liked the product in a general context, weighing up all the other attributes previously evaluated. followed by the frequency of I liked it very much (07) ratings, score 8 and score 7 (03) ratings as shown in graph 5. Graphs 1, 2, 3, 4 and 5 show that the product was well accepted in relation to all the attributes evaluated. It should be noted that none of the evaluators said they disliked any sensory attribute at any level. In the case of the texture attribute, indifference (neither liked nor disliked) was detected, but this represented only 2% of the evaluators, while more than 60% of the evaluators said they liked it very much or not at all. In terms of appearance, color and taste, more than 70% of the evaluators said they liked it very much (score 8) or liked it very much (score 9), the two highest points on the scale used. These results indicate that the cookie produced was well accepted in terms of these attributes. For overall impression, 80% of the evaluators indicated that they liked the product very much. The overall impression expresses how much the evaluator liked the product in a general context, weighing up all the other attributes previously evaluated.

5.3 ACCEPTABILITY INDEX

According to Teixeira et al. (1985), a product with an Acceptability Index (A.I.) of at least 70% has commercial potential. In this sense, it can be seen from Graph 6 that all the sensory quality attributes evaluated obtained an A.I. well above those established in the literature.

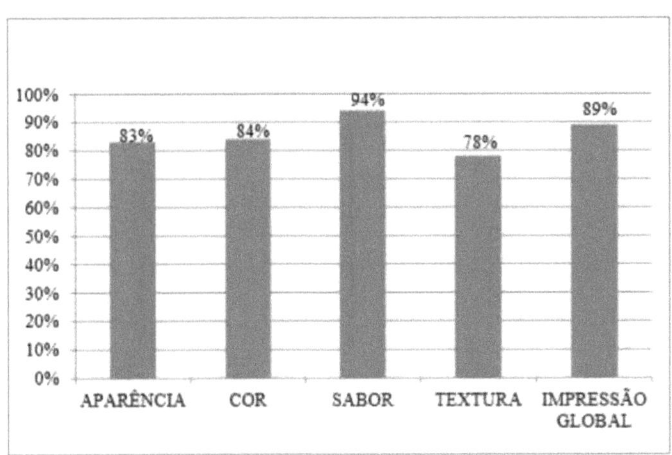

GRAPH 6: Product acceptability indices (Source: Survey data).

Although the tasters did not observe any significant difference in the attributes of the formulation, during the preparation of the product it was seen that the gradual increase in the FBV content correlated with changes in texture, making the product softer and more crumbly. This can be explained by the greater hygroscopicity of the fibrous substances present in green banana flour (FBV), which causes greater water retention, as seen in the study by Silva, Silva, Chang (1998) when they added green banana flour (66%) to cookies. Another technological change observed is related to the color of the formulations. Higher concentrations of FBV promoted a darker color in the samples. This is probably due to the water-retaining capacity of the predominant dietary fiber fractions present in FBV. This retention ends up bringing the molecules closer together and thus concentrating the color of the product (JELTEMA, ZABIK, THIEL, 1983; GUIMARÃES, 2008). It is noteworthy that the process of dehydrating the green banana left the flour with a dark color, characteristic of dehydrated products, quite different from wheat flour, which may also explain the color change in the formulation. It is clear that these changes were discreet and therefore were not perceived by the tasters during the sensory tests. It is noteworthy that the taste attribute obtained an A.I. of 94%, which indicates the product's strong economic potential. Most of the attribute scores were above 7 (I liked it moderately), indicating that the formulation was generally well accepted by the tasters. It is noteworthy that the highest frequency of scores for taste and overall acceptability were 9 (I liked it very much) and 8 (I liked it very much), respectively.

Piovesana et al. (2013), in a study on the acceptability of oat cookies enriched with grape seed flour, concluded that cookies with up to 25% of wheat flour replaced by grape seed flour were well accepted in terms of the sensory attributes evaluated, with an acceptability index of over 70%. These results are in line with those obtained in the present study.

According to Cunha et al. (2010), sensory analysis is a way of translating the consumer's opinion and intention to buy a certain product into numbers, which is why it is so important to verify it in order to really assess the economic potential of the product being offered to the public.

In this way, the preparation was able to fulfill its objective of presenting an easy, practical, low-cost recipe that takes little time to make, as well as encouraging celiacs to produce their own food, using a fruit that is widely found in Brazilian production as a raw material.

These results corroborate studies such as Castillo et al. (2009) and Heisler et al. (2008), which show the feasibility of replacing wheat flour with alternative flours (green banana flour, rice, corn starch, starch, potato starch), obtaining good sensory acceptability.

6 FINAL CONSIDERATIONS

The study is important because of the increase in the number of diagnoses of celiac disease not only in Brazil, but worldwide, making it a public health problem, and given that the only form of treatment currently available is based on removing gluten from the diet. The study showed that it is possible to develop products using green bananas, without compromising product acceptance. The use of green bananas through green banana flour proved to be feasible, since they will be able to consume a product that is widespread in Brazilian production and food, and which has important nutritional characteristics, in addition to its functional properties, providing extra benefits to conventional foods and contributing to greater nutritional, socio-economic and environmental potential. Analysis of the results of the acceptability test led to the conclusion that the methodology used to produce cookies from green banana flour on a laboratory scale was suitable for evaluating the final product. In addition, the good acceptance of the cookies by participants of different age groups made it possible to achieve the main objective of this work, which was to produce a gluten-free food, maintaining its nutritional potential, without compromising its sensory characteristics, and which could be appreciated by the largest number of consumers. Therefore, thanks to the good results obtained in the study, it can be proven that it is possible to use green banana flour in the formulation of a nutritious gluten-free cookie, as an additional alternative on the market, in order to meet the needs of people with celiac disease, without losing the sensory quality of the product.

7 REFERENCES

A. P. **Food bars formulated with soy residues**. Revista Brasileira de Pesquisa em Alimentos. Jul./Dec. 2010, v. 1, n. 2, p. 00-00, Campo Mourao (PR).

ABIMAPI. Brazilian Association of Biscuit, Pasta and Industrialized Bread & Cake Industries. **Cookies**. Available at: http ://www.abimapi.com.br/biscoitos.php. Accessed on December 2, 2016.

ACELBRA - **ASSOCIAÇÃO DOS CELiACOS DO BRASIL**. Statistical data: 2012. Available at: < http://www.acelbra.org.br/2004/index.php>. Accessed on: May 28, 2016

ACELPAR - **Associaçâo dos Celiacos do** Paranà© **2010.** Available at: http://www.acelbra.org.br/2004/dieta.php. Accessed on: December 27, 2016.

ANJO, D. F. C. **Functional** foods **in angiology and vascular surgery.** J Vasc Volume 3, pp. 145-154, 2004.

ANVISA - **National Health Surveillance Agency**. Available at: http://portal.anvisa.gov.br/wps/portal/anvisa/home/. Accessed on: May 28, 2016.

ARAÙJO, H. M. C.; ARAÙJO, W. M. C.; BOTELHO, R. B. A.; ZANDONADI, R. P. **Celiac disease: eating habits and practices and quality of life**. Revista de Nutriçao. Campinas - SP, 2010.

BAPTISTA, M. L. **Celiac disease:** a contemporary view. Available at: http://bases.bireme.br/cgibin/wxislind.exe/iah/online/?IsisScript=iah/iah.xis&src =google&base=LILACS&lang=p&nextAction=lnk&exprSearch=450843&index Search=ID. Accessed on December 2, 2016.

BERNARDES, N. R.; GLÓRIA, L. L.; NUNES, C. R.; PESSANHA, F. F.; MUZITANO, M. F.; OLIVEIRA, D. B. **Quantification of Tannin and Total Phenol Contents and Evaluation of the Antioxidant Activity of Aroeira Fruits.Vértices**, v. 13, p. 117-128, 2011.

BOBBIO, F. O.; BOBBIO, P. A. **Food Processing Chemistry**.

Publisher: Varela - Edition: 3 a. 2001.

BRAZIL . Law No. 10.674, of May 16, 2003. **Obliges commercialized food products to inform about the presence of gluten, as a preventive and control measure for celiac disease**. Official Journal of the Union, Brasilia, DF, May 19, 2003b. p.1.

BRAZIL. Federal Law No. 8,543 of December 23, 1992. **Determines the printing of a warning on labels and packaging of industrialized foods containing gluten, in order to prevent celiac disease**. Official Gazette of the Union of December 24, 1992.

BRIANI C.; SAMAROO D.; ALAEDINI A. **Celiac disease**: from gluten to autoimmunity. Autoimmunity Reviews. 2008

CATASSI, C.; FASANO, A. Celiac disease. **Current Opinion in Gastroenterology,** London, v. 24, n. 6, p. 687-691, 2008.

CÉSAR, A. S.; GOMES, J. C.; SRALIANO, C. D.; FANNI, M. L.; BORGES, M. C. **Elaboration of gluten-free bread**. Revista Ceres, v. 53, n. 306, p. 150-155, 2006.

CESINO, J. M. **Adherence to the gluten-free diet by celiacs in southern Santa Catarina**. Criciùma, 2010.

COBUCCI, R. M. A. **Sensory Analysis**: Course Workbook. Higher Technological Course in Gastronomy. Pontifical Catholic University of Goiás, PUC-GO, 2010.

CRESPO, P. L.; CASTILLEJO G. **Non-dietary therapeutic clinical trials in coeliac disease**. European Journal of Internal Medicine. 2012.

CUNHA, M. A. A.; ANDRADE, A. C. W.; FERMINANI, A. F.; APPELT, P.; BURATTO,

DANTAS, J.L.L.; SOARES FILHO, W.S.; **Botanical classification, origin and evolution**. In: ALVES, E.J.; DANTAS, J.L.L.; SOARES FILHO, W.S.; SILVA, S.O.; OLIVEIRA, M.A.; SOUZA, L.S.; CINTRA, F.L.D.; BORGES, A.L.; OLIVEIRA, A.M.G.; OLIVEIRA, S.L.; FANCELLI, M.; CORDEIRO, Z.J.M.;

SOUZA, J.S. **Banana for export**: technical aspects of production. 2.ed. Brasilia: Embrapa - SPI, 1997, p. 9-13.

DELA LUCIA, S. M. **Statistical methods for evaluating the influence of non-sensory characteristics on consumer acceptance, purchase intensity and choice.** Thesis (Doctorate in Food Science and Technology). Federal University of Viçosa, Viçosa, 2008.

DUTCOSKY, SILVIA D. **Anàlise Sensorial de Alimentos**. 2^a . Ediçao, Curitiba, Editora Champagnat,239 p., 2007.

EL-DASH, A.; GERMANI, R. **Mixed Flour Technology: Use of Mixed Flours in the Production of Biscuits**. EMBRAPA - Empresa Brasileira de Pesquisa Agropecuâria Sistema de Produçao, v. 6, p. 47. Brasilia, 1994.

EMBRAPA. **The banana crop**. Brasilia, DF: Editora Embrapa - SPI, page 910. 1997.

EMBRAPA. Irrigated banana production system. Brasilia, DF: Editora Embrapa - SPI, page 26, 2004.

FAO2011   . FAOSTAR. Available at:

http://faostat.fao.org/site/339/default.aspx. Accessed on: April 10, 2016.

FAO2014   . FAOSTAR. Available at:

http://faostat.fao.org/site/339/default.aspx. Accessed on: April 09, 2016

FASANO A.; CATASSI.; CURRENT C. **Approaches to diagnosis and treatment of celiac disease: an evolving spectrum.** Gastroenterol. 2001

FASOLIN, L. H.; ALMEIDA, G. C. de.; CASTANHO, P. S.; NETTO, E. R. O. **Biscuits produced with banana flour**: chemical, physical and sensory evaluation. Ciênc. Tecnol. Aliment, Campinas, 524-529, 2007.

FASOLIN, L. H.; ALMEIDA, G. C.; CASTANHO, O. S.; NETTO O E R. **Chemical, Physical and sensorial evaluation of banana meal cookies. Ciênc.** Tecnol. Aliment. 787-792, 2007.

FENACELBRA. **National Federation of Celiac Associations of Brazil**. Brasilia, 2013.

FERREIRA, A. **Green Banana: The trendy food. Functional and easy to access**. Available at: https://unibhnutricao.wordpress.com/2014/11/19/1268/. Accessed April 08, 2016.

GIACOBBO L F. **Preparation and characterization of cookies with mixed wheat, soy and green banana flour**. Erechim, 2013.

ADOLFO LUTZ INSTITUTE. **Chemical and physical methods for food analysis.** Sao Paulo, 2008, Chap. IV, p. 98.

ADOLFO LUTZ INSTITUTE. **Chemical and physical methods for food analysis.** Sao Paulo, 2008, Chap. IV, p. 104.

ADOLFO LUTZ INSTITUTE. **Chemical and physical methods for food analysis.** Sao Paulo, 2008, Chap. IV, p. 105.

ADOLFO LUTZ INSTITUTE. **Chemical and physical methods for food analysis.** Sao Paulo, 2008, Chap. IV, p. 123.

ADOLFO LUTZ INSTITUTE. **Normas Analiticas do Instituto Adolfo Lutz.** v. 1: Métodos quimicos e fisicos para análisis de alimentos, 3. ed. Sao Paulo: IMESP, 1985. p. 42-43.

KOHMANN, L.M. **Development of gluten-free white and wholemeal bread fortified with calcium and iron.** Monograph. UFRGS, 2010.

KRUGER, C. L.; MANN, S. W. **Safety evaluation of functional ingredients**. Journal of Food and Chemical Toxicology. Pag 793-805, 2003.

LAJOLO, F, M.; SAURA-CALIXTO, F; WITTING DE PENNA, E.; MENEZES, E, W. **Dietary fiber in Ibero-America:** Technology and health. Origin, characterization, physiological effect and application in food. CYTED XI Project. 6, Obtaining and characterizing dietary fibre for use in special diets. Editora Varela, Sao Paulo, page 469, 2001.

LANGKILDE, A, M.; CHAMP, M.; ANDERSSON, H. **Effects of high-resistant-startch banana flour (RS2) on in vitro fermentation and the smallbowel excretion of energy, nutrients, and sterols:** na ileostomy study. Am J Clin Nutr. V 75, pag 104-111, 2002.

LEFFLER, D. A et al. A **Simple Validated Gluten-Free Diet Adherence Survey for Adults With Celiac Disease. Clinical Gastroenterology and Hepatology,** Volume 7. p 530-536. Available at:

http://www.sciencedirect.com/science/article/pii/S1542356509000081. Accessed on: June 15, 2016.

LERMEN, F. H.; MATIAS, G. S.; MODESTO, F. A.; RODER, R.; BOIKOR, T. J. P. **Consumer testing and analysis of appearance, flavors and colors for the development of new products:** The case of the savored cornbread project. **RELAINEP - Latin American Journal of Innovation and Production Engineering.** Curitiba - PR, v. 3, n. 4, p. 97-109, 2015.

LINDFORS K.; MAKI M.; KAUKINEN K. **Transglutaminase 2-targeted autoantibodies in celiac disease**: Pathogenetic players in addition to diagnostic tools? Autoimmunity Reviews. p.744-9, 2010.

LOBO, A. R. & LEMOS, G. S. M. **Resistant starch and its physico-chemical properties.** Revista Nutrição, Campinas, v. 16, p 219-226, 2003.

MACHADO N C R; SAMPAIO R C. **Effects of resistant starch from green banana biomass.** Trindade, 2013.

MARIA, E, M, P, S.; ATZINGEM, M, C, B, V. **Técnica Dietética Aplicada a Dietoterapia.** Editora Manole pg 03. Barueri - SP, 2005.

MARIANI, M. A. **Physico-chemical and sensory analysis of cookies made with rice flour, rice bran and soy flour as an alternative for celiac patients.** Porto Alegre: Federal University of Rio Grande do Sul - Faculty of Medicine, Degree in Nutrition, 2010.

MEDINA, J. C. **Banana**: culture, raw material, processing and economic aspects.

2nd ed. Campinas: ITAL, 1995.

MINHOTO, M. J. A **brief history of botany**. Available at:

http://botanica.sp.gov.br/. Accessed on: December 26, 2016.

MORAES, C. M. Q. J. **Evaluation of information on the presence or absence of gluten in some industrialized foods**. Rio de Janeiro, 2014.

MORRETO, E.; FETT, R. **Processing and analysis of cookies**. Sao Paulo: Livraria Varela, 1999.

NEUMANN, P., et al. **Healthy foods, functional foods, pharmaceutical foods, nutraceuticals....have you heard of them?** Revista. Hig. Aliment.pag. 19-23, 2002.

NIEWINSKI, M. M. **Advances in celiac disease and gluten-free diet**. Journal of the American Dietetic Association. p.661-72, 2008. Pediatrics. Sao Paulo, 2006.

PEREIRA, A. S.; PEREIRA FILHO, R. **A. Frequent disease, sometimes silent, should be researched and treated**. Available at:

http://www.riosemgluten.com/atualizaca_%20em_DC_silenciosa.htm.   Accessed March 26, 2016.

PEREIRA, K D. **Resistant starch, the latest generation in energy control and healthy digestion**. vol.27, p.88-92, 2007.

PEREZ, P. M. P.; GERMANI, R. **Preparation of savory cookies with high dietary fiber content using eggplant flour (Solanum melongena, L.)**. Revista Ciência e Tecnologia de Alimentos, v. 27, n. 1, p. 186192, 2007

PRATESI R, Gandolfi L. **Celiac disease: an affliction with multiple faces**. 357358, 2006.

PRODANOV, C, C; FREITAS, E, C. **Metodologia do trabalho cientifico: Métodos e técnicas da pesquisa e do trabalho acadêmico**. Available at: https://books.google.com.br/books?hl=pt-BR&lr=&id=zUDsAQAAQBAJ&oi=fnd&pg=PA13&dq=tipos+de+pesquisa+ci entifica&ots=da14fjuayR&sig=9gA88CcXmxuo02o5FYE4okGsZQw#v=onepa

ge&q=tipos%20de%20pesquisa%20cientifica&f=false. Accessed on: June 12, 2016.

RIBEIRO, C. M.; MARTINS, J. F. L.; PAULA, H. A. A.; FERREIRA, C. L. L. F. **Probiotic and technological potential of lactic acid bacteria in the development of** fermented **meat sausages**. Rubio. Rio de Janeiro, 2012

ROBERFROID, M. **Functional food concept and its application to prebiotics**.Editora Elsevier, pag 105. 2002.

RODRIGUES FERREIRA, S. M.; LUPARELLI, P. C.; SCHIEFERDECKER, M. E.; VILELA, R. M. **Gluten-free cookies from sorghum flour**. Archivos Latinoamericanos de Nutrición, Caracas, v. 59, n. 4, p. 433-440, 2009.

SALGADO, S. M.; Faro Z. P.; GUERRA, N. B.; OLIVEIRA, A.V. S. **Physico-chemical aspects of resistant starch**. B. ceppa. 2005

SDEPANIAN, V. *L;* MORAIS, μ. в.; FAGUNDES, N. U. **Celiac disease:** the evolution of knowledge from its original centenary description to the present day. Arquivos de Gastrenterologia. v. 36, n. 4, Oct/Dec. 1999.

SDEPANIAN, V. L.; MORAIS, M. B.; FAGUNDES, N. U. **Celiac disease**: evaluation of compliance with the gluten-free diet and knowledge of the disease by patients registered with the Associaçao dos Celiacos do Brasil (ACELBRA). Sao Paulo, 2001.

SIMABESP. Union of the Pasta and Biscuit Industry in the State of São Paulo: **History of the Biscuit**. Available at:

<http://www.simabesp.org.br/site/historia_biscoito.asp> Accessed December 02, 2016.

SIMMONDS, N.W, SHEPHERD, K. **The taxonomy and origins of the cultivated bananas.** Botanical Journal of the Linnean Society, v.55, p. 302-312, 1955. Abstract available at:

http://onlinelibrary.wiley.com/doi/10.1111/j.1095-8339.1955.tb00015.x/abstract. Accessed December 26, 2016.

SIQUEIRA NETO J. I. et al. **Neurological manifestations of celiac disease**. p. 969-972, 2004. Available

at:http://www.scielo.br/pdf/anp/v62n4/a07v62n4.pdf. Accessed on: June 15, 2016.

SIRÓ, I.; KAPOLNA, E.; KAPOLNA, B.; LUGASI, A. Functional food. Product development, marketing and consumer acceptance - A review. Appetite, Volume 51, Hungary, pages 456-467, 2008.

SOUZA, P. H. M.; SOUZA NETO, M. H.; MAIA, G. A. **Functional components in food**. Boletim da SBCTA. v. 37, n. 2, p. 127-135, 2003.

TAIPINA, M. S.; FONTS, M. A. S.; COHEN, V. H. **Functional foods - nutraceuticals. Food Hygiene**. v. 16, n. 100, p 28-29, 2002.

TEIXEIRA, E.; MEINERT, E.M.; BARBETTA, P.A. **Análise sensorial de alimentos**. Florianópolis: Editora da UFSC, 1985.

TEIXEIRA, L. V. **Sensory analysis in the food industry.** Revista do Instituto de Laticinios Càndido Tostes, v. 64, n. 366, p. 12-21, 2009.

THOMPSON, T.; DENNIS, M.; HIGGINS, L.A.; LEE, A.R.; SHARRETT, M.K. **Gluten-fre siet survey**: are the Americans with celiac disease consuming recommended amounts of fibre, iron, calcium and grain foods? The British Dietetic Association LTDA. Journal of Human Nutrition Dietetic. p. 163-169, 2005.

VALLE, H. F; CAMARGOS M. **Yes, we have bananas:** stories and recipes with green banana biomass. Editora Senac. Sao Paulo, 2003.

VAN DOKKUM, W. **Functional properties of dietary fiber, resistant starch and non-digestible oligosaccharides**. Viçosa, 2008.

VASCONCELLOS F; CAVALCANTE E; BARBOSA L. **Menu**: how to put together an efficient menu. Sao Paulo: Roca, 2002.

WALZEM, R. L. **Functional Foods.** Trends in Food Science and Technology. pag. 518, 2004.

ZANDONADI, R. R. **Green banana pasta**: an alternative for gluten exclusion.

Thesis (Doctorate in Health Sciences), Faculty of Health Sciences, University of Brasilia - UnB, Brasilia, 2009.

ZHANG, P.; WAMPLER, J, L.; BRUNIA, A, K.; BURKHOLDER, K, M.; PATTERSON, J, A.; WHISTLER, R, L. **Effects of arabinoxylans on activation of mrine macrophages and growth performace of broiler chicks**. Cereal Chemistry. V 81, p 511-514, 2005.

ZHANG, P.; WHISTLER, R. L.; BEMILLER, J.N.; HAMAKER, B. R. **Banana starch:** production, physicochemical properties, and digestibility. Caboidrate Polymers, West Lafayette, v. 59, p. 443-458, 2005.

ZUCCO, F.; BORSUK, Y.; ARNTFIELD, S. D. Physical and nutritional evaluation of wheat cookies supplemented with pulse flours of different particle sizes. **LWT - Food Science and Technology**, Campinas, v. 44, n. 10, p. 20702076, 2011.

APPENDIX A - ACCEPTABILITY QUESTIONNAIRE

MAURICIO DE NASSAU COLLEGE

FAP UNIT - PARNAÎBA

COURSE: BACHELOR OF NUTRITION

AcEITABILITY TEST

Name: _______________________________________ Date: _____ // ___

Sex: Female (   ) Male (   ) Age: _______

You will receive a tasting sample which will be served individually.
 Try it carefully and rate it according to the scale below.

DO YOU HAVE AN ALLERGY TO BRAZIL NUTS?

Name of the product: <u>Gluten-free *cookie* made from green banana flour</u>

9 - I liked it a lot

8 - I liked it a lot

7 - I liked it moderately

6 - I liked it slightly

5 - Neither liked nor disliked

4 - Slightly disliked

3 - Moderately disliked

2 - I really dislike it

1 - I really dislike it

Appearance	Color	Flavor	Texture	Global Print

Comments: ____

Thank you for your participation!

APPENDIX B - INFORMED CONSENT FORM

I, **MARIA JANETE GOMES RIBEIRO**, student of Nutrition at Faculdade Mauricio de Nassau - Unidade FAP Parnaiba, have developed a study for the Course Conclusion Work (TCC II) entitled "BISCOITO COOKIE FROM GREEN BANANA FLOUR: An alternative for people with celiac disease". You You will be informed that by participating in this project, you will be taking part in an academic study, the aim of which is to research the cookie produced from green banana flour as an alternative for people with celiac disease.

Although you have agreed to take part in this project, you are guaranteed that you can withdraw at any time by simply informing us of your decision. You will also be informed that, as this is a voluntary participation, you will not be entitled to any remuneration. There will be no risk or harm to your health. Your data will be kept confidential, as guaranteed by Resolution 196/96 of the National Health Council (CNS), and you will be able to request information during the research, including after the publication of the data obtained from it.

Parnaiba (PI)de 2016.

Me, .

I have been informed about the survey BISCOITO COOKIE A

FROM GREEN BANANA FLOUR: An alternative for people with celiac disease. I agree to participate voluntarily and consent to my data being used in the study.

Participant's signature: ____

Signature of researcher: _______________________________

ANNEXES

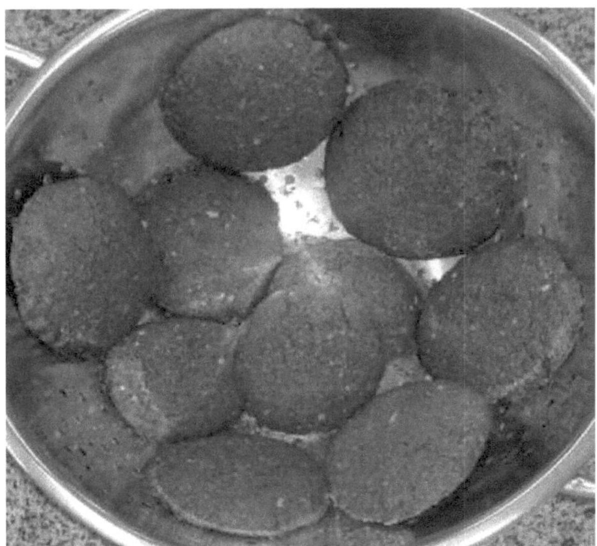

Figure 1: *Cookie* made with green banana flour

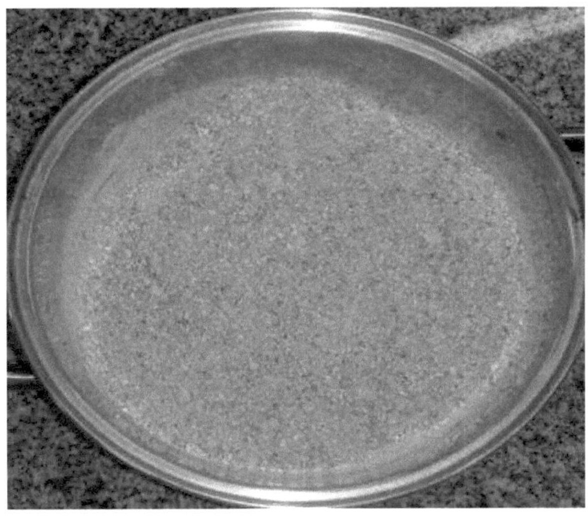

Figure 2: Green banana flour

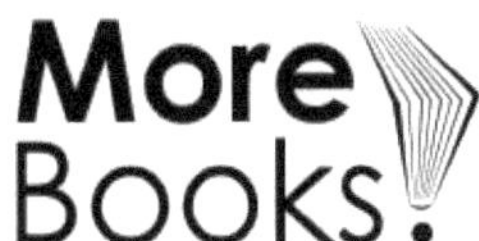

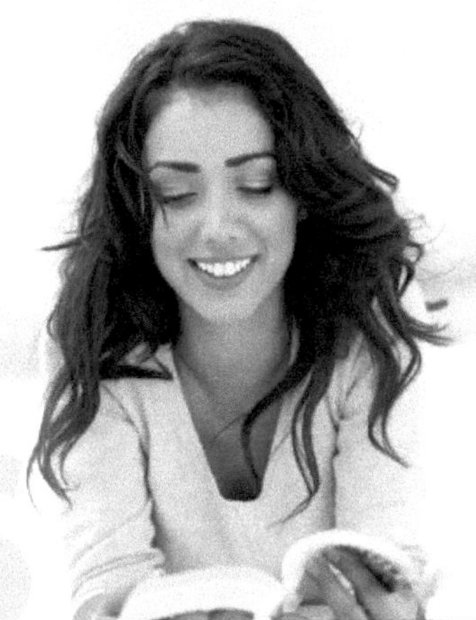

I want morebooks!

Buy your books fast and straightforward online - at one of world's fastest growing online book stores! Environmentally sound due to Print-on-Demand technologies.

Buy your books online at
www.morebooks.shop

Kaufen Sie Ihre Bücher schnell und unkompliziert online – auf einer der am schnellsten wachsenden Buchhandelsplattformen weltweit! Dank Print-On-Demand umwelt- und ressourcenschonend produziert.

Bücher schneller online kaufen
www.morebooks.shop

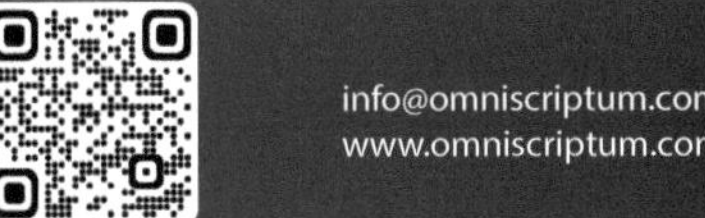

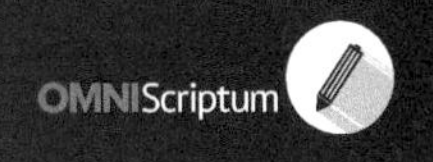

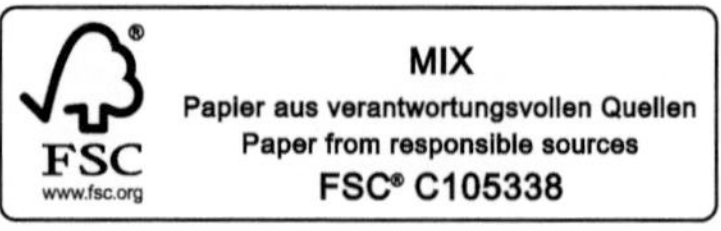

Printed by Books on Demand GmbH, Norderstedt / Germany